The
Diabetes Cure

What you need to know about diabetes: diet,
cure and solution for life

Table of Contents

Introduction 1

Chapter 1: Understanding Diabetes 2

Chapter 2: Common Misconceptions 8

Chapter 3: How to Test for Diabetes 12

Chapter 4: Diet 17

Chapter 5: Physical Activity 21

Chapter 6: Cure and Solution 25

Bonus Chapter: Staying Positive 31

Conclusion 33

Introduction

I want to thank you and congratulate you for downloading the book, "The Diabetes Cure: What you need to know about diabetes: diet, cure and solution for life".

This is the book that will tell you all the basic things that you need to know about diabetes and the things that you can do to make sure that you can continue living a wonderful life.

Don't feel hopeless because there is a way that you can take full control of your body and your disease and this book will show you how.

Some individuals feel hopeless about their current situation. However, the fact is that diabetes can be managed.

It will take some effort to make the necessary changes but there is a good chance that you can still live a good life in spite of this condition.

You will just have to incorporate little changes in your diet and physical activities and be obedient enough to listen to what your doctor tells you.

This book also provides tips on how to alleviate the symptoms; and if you can be successful, even prevent the symptoms from occurring again.

With the guidelines provided in this this book, and with the help of your doctor, you will have a different mindset about your condition and look forward to days of fruitful activities.

Thanks again for downloading this book, I hope you enjoy it!

CHAPTER 1

Understanding Diabetes

If there's anything that you need to understand deeply about your body, it should be how it produces insulin, the enzyme that causes the breaking down of carbohydrates into utilizable components.

The pancreas is the organ that manufactures insulin.

Back in your elementary or high school days, you might have been taught about the function of carbohydrates in our body. They are the providers of energy. Without carbohydrates, you will feel tired or weak.

In the absence of sufficient amount of carbohydrates, your body will utilize protein coming from your muscles for energy. You can become thin because of this.

Your doctor will determine the carbohydrate utilization mode your body is using. One mode is that your pancreas is unable to produce enough insulin.

The other mode is where it is able to produce the enzyme but the kind of insulin that is produced is not effective in breaking down carbohydrates (which includes the sugars that you eat).

Unprocessed carbohydrates just remain in the blood until they are flushed out in the urine. This increased amount of carbohydrates/sugar in the blood compels the body to flush out water frequently.

This is the reason why diabetics visit the toilet more frequently than before. And when they do that, the immediate consequence is the body will lack fluids.

That's why you always get thirsty. These are the three observable symptoms of diabetes – tiredness, frequent urination and thirstiness.

There are three main types of diabetes – Type 1 diabetes, Type 2 diabetes, and Gestational diabetes.

The three types of diabetes are characterized by an unusually high level of blood sugar. This is either because the body cannot produce sufficient insulin or cannot use the insulin produced, or sometimes even both.

Insulin as mentioned earlier is the hormone needed by the cells in the body to take up glucose, which is needed for energy.

High levels of blood sugar can lead to damage in the tiny blood vessels in the kidneys, heart, eyes, or nervous system.

Diabetes may therefore lead to cardiovascular diseases, kidney diseases, vision impairment and blindness, as well as damage to the nervous system, if left undetected and untreated.

Type 1 diabetes

Type 1 diabetes is also called insulin-dependent diabetes. It is a condition where insulin production is absent because the immune system of the body attacks the beta cells of the pancreas that produce insulin.

No one has yet established the reason why this happens. Type 1 diabetes may possibly be triggered by environmental factors and genetic predispositions.

Some experts assume that there are abnormal reactions happening in those cells, which are caused by some bacteria or viruses such as the Epstein-Barr virus and retroviruses. Diet is also considered another factor.

Some studies find an increased risk of Type 1 diabetes in infants due to exposure to cow's milk, high nitrate concentration in potable water, and low exposure to vitamin D.

In very rare cases, diabetes results from diseases that attack the pancreas.

Type 1 diabetes usually develops in childhood or adolescence; hence, it was formerly called juvenile-onset diabetes.

However, due to the emergence of this type of diabetes in other age groups, the terms using age of onset are no longer accurate.

Several medical risks are linked to Type 1 diabetes.

Aside from the serious risk of cardiovascular diseases and stroke, damage can occur in the blood vessels of the eyes (diabetic retinopathy), in the nerves (diabetic neuropathy), and in the kidneys (diabetic nephropathy).

It is common that individuals will blame diabetes symptoms on "overworking" or "getting older," butthese are misguided beliefs, of course.

Anyone can have diabetes. When we talk about diabetes, we need to prevent it.

Prevention is always better than cure. And hence, it is absolutely necessary to screen for the disease if one is at a great risk for it. Earlier detection can prevent serious diabetes complications.

For Type 1 diabetes, the symptoms develop very quickly and show in a matter of weeks.

The symptoms may initially be mistaken for flu or similar illnesses. Individuals with Type 1 diabetes exhibit the following symptoms:

- Frequent urination – This may be all the more observable during night-time when the kidneys work extra hard to flush out the excess sugar in the blood. This is accompanied by flushing out more water. Urination therefore gets rid of excess sugar and water. Doing it frequently indicates a high blood sugar level.
- Insatiable thirst – The more water you lose through urination or sweating, the more dehydrated the cells in your body become. Frequent urination will dehydrate the body

faster and cause thirstiness in a person. Dehydration may lead to dry skin and parched mouths.

- Unexplained weight loss – This may occur due to dehydration or when all of the sugar in the blood is flushed out in urine instead of being used for energy by the cells of the body.
- Increased hunger – which follows when the calories supposed to be used by the body for energy is flushed out in the urine instead.
- Changes in the vision – Blurriness may occur as a result of sugar build-up in the lens of the eyes incurring a change in lens shape.
- Lethargy – Feeling weak, tired and unenthusiastic about accomplishing things all the time follows when blood sugar, which provides the energy to be used by the body is not utilized, but rather expelled out of the system through urination.

Type 2 diabetes

Type 2 diabetes is also called non-insulin-dependent diabetes. In this type of diabetes, the pancreas produces insulin; however, the amount is either not sufficient for the needs of the body, or the body's cells resist it.

This is called insulin resistance. It occurs usually in fat, liver and the muscle cells. Insulin resistance causes the pancreas to overly produce insulin to bring about an effect. Still, the blood sugar remains very high.

Type 2 diabetes is the most common type of diabetes. Seventy-five percent of diabetics around the world suffer from this type of diabetes.

This type of diabetes is prevalent in those with African-Caribbean descent, in American Indians, in Hispanics and in South Asian. However, the expression of this condition cannot be tied down to a single gene. Obesity and weight gain are also important determinants of Type 2 diabetes.

Type 2 diabetes, in comparison to Type 1 diabetes is milder.

Still, it can lead to major health problems affecting the blood vessels of the kidneys, nerves, and eyes. It can also lead to cardiovascular diseases and stroke.

It used to be called adult-onset diabetes as it commonly appears among individuals who are in their middle ages, but it can also be developed in younger individuals who possess the following characteristics:

- With a history of diabetes in their family
- Are overweight or obese
- Live a sedentary lifestyle
- Have already experienced heart attack, hypertension or stroke
- Have heart disease or high blood pressure
- Have been determined to have a marginal blood glucose examination result
- Overweight women who have been diagnosed to be suffering from polycystic ovary syndrome
- Women diagnosed with high level of blood glucose during pregnancy (gestational diabetes)

Symptoms of Type 2 diabetes are slow to show, usually appearing at later stages in life, by which time serious health complications may have already occurred. The longer it remains undetected and untreated, the greater is the severity of organ damage.

Some individuals will only discover the problem through a routine medical examination. Preventive measures must be taken to reduce the risk of developing this type of diabetes and its complications.

Apart from the above-mentioned symptoms of Type 1 diabetes, those with Type 2 diabetes may express fainting, headaches, numbness and tingling of the extremities, and in rare cases, loss of consciousness.

They may also have several yeast-induced infections. Another symptom is itching around the vagina or groin.

Skin color may darken around the neck, armpits and crotch areas. Careful observation must be givento slow-healing sores or cuts, especially those in the feet.

If you have slow-healing wounds in the feet, this is cause for immediate concern. Contact your doctor immediately.

Gestational diabetes

The third type of diabetes is Gestational diabetes. It is often diagnosed during the middle or late stage of pregnancy.

As the blood circulates through the placenta of the mother to the baby, important care must be taken to control blood sugar level as high levels may negatively affect the growth and development of the baby.

Gestational diabetes affects both the mother and the baby. A caesarean section may be needed due to an overly large baby. It can also affect the heart, kidney, nerves and eyes of the mother.

Moreover, it puts the mother at a greater risk for developing Type 2 diabetes, anywhere from a few weeks after delivery to months or years later.

Risks to the baby include abnormal weight gain before birth, breathing problems at birth, obesity and diabetes risk later in life.

CHAPTER 2

Common Misconceptions

There are misconceptions about the other causes of diabetes and the most prominent one among them is the belief that eating sweet foods in large amounts can cause diabetes. This is only partly true.

One of the major risk factors for developing diabetes is obesity. Eating sweet foods in excessive amounts can lead to obesity, which in turn may contribute to diabetes.

However, diabetes can develop even in individuals who avoid sweet foods. This can be attributed to other risk factors for diabetes which include age, family history of diabetes and sedentary lifestyle.

The belief that only obese individuals get diabetes is false. As a matter of fact, anyone can develop diabetes.

However, individuals who are obese or overweight are at a greater risk of developing the condition. About 25% of patients who develop Type 2 diabetes in the US are not obese.

It is also a common misconception to associate diabetes with old age.

While it is true that the largest group of patients diagnosed with diabetes comprises of individuals aged 65 years and older, individuals across all age groups can be diagnosed with diabetes including children and young adults.

Due to undiagnosed cases, even those who have no family history of diabetes can develop diabetes. However, there is an increased risk of developing diabetes for those who have diabetic first-degree or second-degree relatives.

Many people strongly believe that diabetes manifests in signs and symptoms. So until they really see or feel these, there is no reason for actual concern.

In truth, for many diabetics, most of the signs and symptoms occur only after serious complications have set in. The longer diabetes remains undetected and untreated, the greater is the severity of organ damage.

There are about 387 million patients around the world who are struggling with diabetes. It is estimated that nearly one third of individuals with diabetes are unaware that they have this condition.

It is therefore important to screen for the condition if you possess any of the characteristics mentioned earlier.

Some individuals deliberately refuse a screening even if they possess some or all of the characteristics mentioned earlier. They fear that diabetics need to take medicine constantly for life. This is false as not all diabetics need medication. Some of them may be able to use diet and exercise alone to control their blood sugar.

Some also avoid screening as they believe a diagnosis of the condition includes a permanent restriction on starchy food such as bread, potatoes and pasta.

All these can be part of a well-balanced diet that is necessary to help keep the blood sugar at a normal range.

Even small amounts of pleasurable confectionery such as sweets and chocolates are allowed for diabetics, with the advice of their doctor and dietician. It all boils down to moderation and meal portions.

Those who are at risk of diabetes fear that being diagnosed of the condition would mean they can no longer partake in sports or leisure activities that require physical exertion. They fear that they will tire easily at work.

In fact, the opposite is true. A key role in the management of diabetes is regular physical exercise. Diabetics can take inspiration from several top-performing athletes who happen to be diabetic.

However, these individuals should build the discipline to calculate and time food intake and medication to prevent low blood sugar.

With the help of a doctor, they can plot a proper schedule that does not put them in a situation where they do more harm to their body on account of their physical activities.

There are several ways to manage or treat diabetes such that it does not prevent someone from the life he or she is already leading.

Managing diabetes simply means keeping blood sugar in a normal range, so that one does not experience its associated symptoms or cause internal damage to the body organs. This will include a lifestyle modification and medication if necessary.

Diabetic patients who are advised to take medication fear that they will need frequent injections to maintain their blood sugar.

Not all patients actually require injected insulin. Only about 25% of diabetic patients use insulin in the US. Others take oral medication as advised by their doctors.

There is no absolute claim that non-traditional methods such as herbal remedies can cure diabetes.

While some scientific studies show that certain herbal remedies may manage diabetes, others in contrast show that these may cause unwanted side effects and interfere with doctor-prescribed medications. It's always best to consult a doctor before using such supplements.

Some think that stress is another cause.

This is not true either, but stress can worsen the symptoms. Accidents and illnesses may show that someone has been harboring the diabetes, but no, these things do not cause diabetes.

Remember that diabetes is non-communicable. Diabetes cannot be caught like a cold or flu. There is no way that a victim can pass it to anyone. Neither is one more likely to get a cold or another illness if he or she is diabetic.

However, individuals with diabetes are advised to get flu shots.

This is necessary because any illness can complicate the condition of diabetes, making it more difficult to control and manage. Individuals with diabetes who contract the flu often tend to develop more serious complications than others.

CHAPTER 3

How to Test for Diabetes

It is important that you realize that there's something that you can do to alleviate the problem.

The more you know about your condition, the more possible it is that you can lead a healthy life, live the life that you want to live and avoid the complications that are associated with the disease.

For all types of diabetes, the symptoms can be easily relieved once you get the proper treatment. Early treatment can also help in avoiding serious complications.

It is good that you are aware that you have the disease, because many individuals don't. For one person who knows that he has the disease, there's another one who doesn't know. The disease rarely occurs in infants.

If you possess some or all of the characteristics mentioned in the first chapter that put you at a greater risk for diabetes, you must approach a doctor for advice. If he or she deems you at risk, you may be asked to undergo blood tests that may be repeated to confirm results.

There are three ways to get blood tested for diabetes- Fasting Blood Glucose and Oral Glucose Tolerance Test.

Fasting Blood Glucose is the more common test, wherein the patient is asked to fast for 8 hours before blood is extracted to measure blood sugar.

If the test result exceeds the normal range, the doctor might consider a diagnosis of diabetes, based on the patient's other risk factors or symptoms. A repeat test is usually conducted to confirm the result.

The Oral Glucose Tolerance Test is more definitive. It is given to patients with borderline or no definitive results in Fasting Blood Glucose.

The patient is asked to drink a sugar solution. Thereafter, several blood extractions are taken in order to evaluate how his or her system responds to the sugar.

A third test, the Hemoglobin A1C test is a blood test that estimates average glucose levels in the blood over the past three to four months.

Periodic Hemoglobin A1C testing is conducted to see how well diet, exercise, and medications are working to control blood sugar and prevent organ damage.

Some individuals are not diabetic, but are instead pre-diabetic.

Prediabetes is the condition when blood glucose levels are high, but not high enough to qualify as diabetes.

It may however lead to diabetes in 10 years or lower. Just like diabetics, pre-diabetics have a higher risk of heart disease and stroke.

Prediabetes may lead to diabetes if left uncontrolled, which may result to either minor or obvious organ damage depending on how long the disease goes undetected. The longer diabetes goes undetected and untreated, the more serious is the damage to organs.

Pre-diabetics can delay or prevent the development of diabetes through a lifestyle change wherein they are asked to lose weight and increase physical activity. Medication is also prescribed.

It is better to screen early for diabetes as early detection allows doctors to prescribe the right treatments to decrease the risk of further complications and more serious organ damage.

Once diagnosed with diabetes, the doctor will evaluate the extent and severity of any damage done to the organs.

As mentioned in earlier chapters, diabetes primarily affects the heart and blood vessels, kidneys, eyes and nerves. After evaluating the extent of the disease, the doctor will create a plan. A plan is vital to control the patient's blood sugar at all times.

It is important for one to fully cooperate with his or her doctor to come up with an effective plan to manage diabetes.

It's easier to think of the doctor as a friend and as someone who wants only what's best for the patient.

Walls need to come down and trust needs to be built between the doctor and patient.

With the doctor's help in creating a proper plan, one can live an active, full, and happy life even with diabetes which is a life-long, but manageable condition.

The doctor will ask the patient several questions to get accurate information. A lot can be revealed from one's family history, so the patient must be ready to answer to the best of his or her knowledge.

This will make it easier for the doctor to better understand the condition and make an effective plan thereafter. It is perfectly all right to ask the doctor to repeat questions to clarify.

It is completely understandable to forget all the symptoms one has experienced before scheduling a visit to the doctor.

If this happens, there is no harm in bringing this up on the next visit. In the same way, it is advisable to make a mental note of experiences in between visits.

Describing the circumstances around those experiences will give a complete picture of the condition. Mention these to the doctor, so that everything is taken into account when creating an effective diabetes plan.

As part of the evaluation, the patient may be advised to undergo several tests apart from blood tests that may include ultrasound or x-ray tests, as well as challenge tests. It is better to bring along old test results, so these can be compared with the current results.

Upon the doctor's evaluation, lifestyle changes, possible medication, and periodic blood glucose testing may be prescribed, all with the primary goal of keeping the blood sugar under control.

Depending on the type and extent of the diabetes, medication may be prescribed which can be either the oral or injectable type. However, if a patient experiences side effects or has problems with the medication, it's best to inform the doctor immediately.

Lifestyle modification will include changes in the diet, increase in physical activities, as well as stopping altogether unhealthy habits like smoking.

There may be many changes in lifestyle which can be discussed in detail with the doctor, should the patient find difficulty in following these.

Remember, to be able to manage diabetes, one will need to start changing certain things in life.

These aren't meant to hamper happiness, but rather ensure that one can live a full and active life even with this life-long condition.

The patient will also be referred to a dietician who will help prepare specialized meal plans and demonstrate how to better develop a well-balanced meal to keep the blood sugar within a normal range.

If a patient has religious or personal concerns, these may be discussed with the dietician who will take these into account when creating the specialized meal plans.

Remember again, that being diabetic doesn't mean eating foods that are different from the ones eaten by those who are not afflicted by the condition. It all comes down to portions and eating in moderation.

Creating a diabetes plan is only the start of diabetes management.

A patient must be committed to it. By sticking to the plan, he or she can keep blood sugar within a normal range, thereby preventing further complications.

The patient will need to track his or her progress by monitoring blood sugar daily. Keeping a diary is advisable so the patient can take down blood sugar readings and the time when the readings were taken.

Also include diet and activities in the diary, so that it's easy to report to the doctor with accuracy on the next visit.

CHAPTER 4

Diet

Make changes in your lifestyle. Eat healthy foods. In particular, avoid foods that can increase the level of glucose in your blood.

Your meals, though, should not look different from those that individuals without diabetes eat.

The only caveat is that you should make sure to eat foods that are low in sugar, fat and salt.

Meals should contain some starchy foods, vegetables and fruits.

Coming up with healthy meals should not be troublesome.

You can actually have foods that taste great. If you need guidance, your doctor can recommend a dietitian. For the meantime, here is a quick guide for you.

- Eat foods that have low glycemic index (GI) and those that have nutrients which typical western meals lack. Experts suggest eating foods high in calcium, fiber, magnesium, potassium, and vitamins A, C and E. Fiber has the ability to help the body avoid constipation and lower cholesterol and blood glucose levels. It is also a must that you supply your body with a lot of vitamins and mineral through the foods that you eat, especially the water-soluble ones. You are frequently urinating and that means you are losing substantial amounts of water-soluble nutrients in your urine.

  Beans are a good source of fiber, potassium and magnesium. You can have black beans, navy beans, pinto beans and kidney beans.

If you've got enough of beans for 1 day, a third of your daily fiber requirement is already met.

In addition, eating one-half cup of beans can provide you protein with the amount that an ounce of meat can provide. You can buy canned beans for convenience and for saving time.

Always include green leafy vegetables such as kale, spinach and collards. This is the surest way to cut down on calories.

For the same purpose, have citrus fruits. Limes, lemons, grapefruit, oranges and many others can give lots of Vitamin C and fiber also.

Tomatoes are also good sources of Vitamin C. However you want your tomatoes – pureed or raw –you'll get a good supply of iron and Vitamin E.

Replace your regular potatoes with sweet potatoes and you can get large amounts of Vitamin A. Sweet potatoes are some of the best foods to eat for low glycemic index.

For antioxidants, have lots of berries. Antioxidants are said to be able to improve the reaction of the cells to insulin.

Whole grains, like oatmeal and pearled barley, are very beneficial to you. They contain potassium, fiber, folate, omega 3 fatty acids, chromium and magnesium.

Don't buy processed grains like the ones that you get from bread. You must eat bran and germ from whole grains in their most natural state.

Have some nuts because they can help in the management of your hunger. They also provide healthy fats and omega 3 fatty acids. Eat plenty of flax seeds and walnuts.

- Your regular meals should be based on foods that are starchy. Add cereals, pasta and potatoes to control your blood glucose to your meals. Whole grains must always be there in your meals.

- As a diabetic, you are prone to developing heart disease. With that in mind, always make sure that you minimize eating fatty foods. In particular, be wary of saturated fats. Among the top 10 foods high in saturated fats are hydrogenated oil, desiccated coconut, butter, animal fats, chocolates, fish oils, cheese, and ice cream. To make sure that you are really cutting down on fats, do the following:
  1. Eat dairy foods that are really low in fat. Examples are skimmed milk, yoghurt and custard.
  2. Pick lean meats such as skinless chicken. Get rid of all visible fatty parts before cooking.
  3. Cut down on frying foods. Opt for cooking procedures that do not use oil. You can do microwaving, grilling, barbecuing, poaching, steaming and dry roasting instead.
  4. When cooking, scoop away the oils from the top of curries, stews and casseroles.
  5. It's time to throw away the oils that you regularly use. Use instead, rapeseed, ground nut and olive oils.
  6. Packing your refrigerator and tables with fruits and vegetables is a good way to shy away from foods that contain harmful oils. Have five portions of them in one day. Think about incorporating fruits and vegetables during your snack time. There are no limits for you when it comes to these types of foods. You can eat all kinds of fruits and vegetables.
- Abhor sugary foods. They are the reasons why you sometimes feel nauseous. This is because sugary foods can make your glucose levels drastically rise up. However, there is no need to completely do away with sugars. Just avoid drinks and snack foods that are too sweet. You can have sugar-free squash and diet drinks, for instance.
- You are also prone to developing high blood pressure. Cut down on salt consumption and drink a lot of water. Avoid any type of salty food to stay on the safe side. You may try spices as alternatives to salt. For instance, instead of adding salt to a hardboiled egg, use pepper and other spices instead. Some diabetics look for processed foods that don't

use too much salt. If possible, always eat natural and non-processed foods. The following foods are to be avoided:

- Boxed mixes of rice, pasta and potatoes
- Canned meats, vegetables, soups and sauces
- Processed foods
- Spreads, salad dressings, mustard, gravies, ketchup and pickled foods
- Ham, bacon, sausage and luncheon meat
- Salty snack foods
- msg
- Soy sauce and steak sauce

• Alcohol isn't completely prohibited, but make sure that you don't get intoxicated. Check with your doctor if you are even allowed to use it because alcohol can trigger a drastic rise in blood sugar. Alcohol also contains a lot of calories.

For women with diabetes, allowable amount is two units while for men three units. A unit is equivalent to a glass of wine or a half pint of beer. For spirits, take no more than 25 ml per day.

Alcohol can increase your appetite, so you may overeat and cause your blood sugar to rise. It can also interfere with the actions and effects and oral medicines you are taking.

Make it a point to lose weight if overweight, but keep in mind to be gradual in doing it.

Crash dieting is a big no-no for individuals with diabetes. This is because it is also harmful for you to severely lower your blood glucose.

Individuals with normal body weight can easily control their glucose levels.

CHAPTER 5

Physical Activity

Focus on improving your physical activities.

Living a more active lifestyle can help regulate glucose levels, reducing weight, avoiding heart diseases, regulate blood pressure and blood cholesterol levels, and make insulin work effectively.

Surprisingly, being more active will result to feeling less exhausted and stressed.

Create a plan towards this aim and you should have a definite goal. Come up with a set of rewarding, safe and fun-to-do routines.

Making routines fun and enjoyable is very important. Remember that you will need a lot of encouragement.

If your workouts and exercise routines are fun, you will do them on your own.

You will do them without being prodded by those who care for you.

Make sure also that the physical activities will not compromise your safety, particularly avoiding those that can cause you injuries and soreness in your muscles. Accidents and injuries can just cause you to lose motivation.

It is important that you get inputs from your doctor and other members of your health care team when planning your routine.

They will discuss the desired target range for your blood glucose levels with you. If your glucose level goes very low due to excessive movements, you may develop hypoglycemia, which is also very dangerous.

Some individuals pass out, go into a coma, or experience seizures because of hypoglycemia. Your team will tell you how to avoid that. Ask them for changes needed in your exercise routine and other physical activities.

In most cases, health care teams impose changes in diet and medications for diabetic patients who engage in physically demanding or strenuous exercises. Again, the aim is to keep your blood glucose levels within the target range.

Before starting, make sure that you have already identified the days of the week and the time of the day for your workout, the duration of each session, your warming exercises, stretching, and exercises for cooling down.

You should also plan the alternative activities that you can do when original workouts you had in mind cannot be used.

You should also plan how you will keep track of your progress. Take notes of your blood glucose levels before and after doing any strenuous activities.

The length of time of each workout or repetition and the amount of heavy lifting you're going to do are the two things you should record. Prepare a notebook for record keeping purposes.

After taking down notes for about seven days, you should have an idea of which are the best activities that can help you maintain the right levels and how long they should be done in a given session.

Pick one or two friends or relatives to be your exercise buddy. You will find that it is easier and more fun to do physical activities when somebody is joining you.

What are good activities for you? The rule of thumb is to do something that you really enjoy doing.

For example, you can start with walking to the park and back to your home. Gardening early in the morning is also good.

These are activities which you can habitually do because they are easy to perform.

Start with something that you can do continuously for 30 minutes. If in the beginning, you feel you just cannot do the same activity for that length of time, do it for less than 10 minutes.

There are other things that you can do throughout the day to compensate. Just remember to always be on the move and try to avoid the computer and TV. At home, you can always make use of the stairs.

Program your house work. When traveling, make plans to leave your house early. With time at your side, you can have the luxury of getting off a train or bus one station earlier. Then you can take a walk to your destination.

Always enjoy the scenery while walking. Individuals like you must take every opportunity to calm your mind and enjoy the best things that life can offer.

You will find walking as the easiest activity to do, but you will have to level up from this type. Diabetic individuals are encouraged to have light activities, then the moderate ones and finally, heavy or vigorous types.

If you can normally breathe or talk after doing an activity for 30 minutes, you can categorize it as light. If you are gasping for breath and are sweating after about 10 minutes, mark it as a moderate type.

Intense activities are those that can make you breathe deeply. With that type, you might not be able to talk normally without pausing to take a breath first.

You must learn how to correctly categorize activities because, remember, you are taking down notes and those notes must give you precise measurements.

The notes are your guide on how your body responds to different kinds of physical activities. For the heavy ones,, you can try golfing, dancing, tennis, cycling and swimming.

Increase movements while making effort to change the way you do your daily chores and tasks.

When talking with someone over the phone, don't sit on a chair. Move around. When watching TV, stand up and do some cleaning in the room during advertisements.

Lengthen the time that you do your house chores. For instance, you can take two trips instead of one when taking soiled clothes to the laundry room.

When parking the car, park a little farther from your destination. Use the stairs rather than the elevator.

Change the way you think about breaks. From now on, your break times are opportunities to move about and looking at the sceneries you probably have never noticed before.

Walk around or do muscle stretching. To be unmoving is your biggest enemy.

Wherever you intend to do your physical activities, always bring starchy carbohydrate (a sandwich for example), glucose tablets or some sweets.

This is more especially being advised to those who are receiving insulin injections or ingesting sulfonylurea tablets.

Just in case your blood glucose levels get too low and you experience dizziness because of the extra activities, immediately gobble some of these. The ideal level for blood glucose is 4-6 mmol/l before a meal and 10 mmol/l after a meal.

The circumference of your waist is a good indicator of your progress. For men, the goal is trim it down to 94 cm, but for Asian men, the ideal circumference is 90. For all women, it should be 80 cm.

If you are being treated with insulin injections, make sure that your physical activities don't involve too much the injection site.

It is not good for you to do cycling if your leg is the injection site. Discuss with your doctor the need to change the injection site if you really get pleasure from using a bike.

Chapter 6

Cure and Solution

Is there a cure for diabetes? Unfortunately, there is currently no known cure. With all the advancements and research towards developing one, medical science has not yet discovered an effective treatment to stop diabetes for both types.

This means you will have to live all your days with the disease. But then again, you don't have to be miserable. Your key is proper management. Relax, avoid stress, eat a balanced diet, and get proper exercise.

Despite the absence of an ultimate cure, there are various treatments, both natural and medical. Natural supplements for diabetes are available, but you need to be careful about using them.

Even natural substances can adversely affect your medications and the chemical reactions of the body.

There are good news coming from some individuals who have used these supplements, but still, always consult with your doctor before buying and using.

Emotional stress has been shown to increase blood glucose levels, so make sure that you work towards gaining a peaceful mind and heart.

You may try non-conventional natural therapies such as acupuncture, guided imagery, biofeedback, progressive muscle relaxation and deep abdominal breathing.

Acupuncture is non-conventional therapy that makes use of thin needle insertions in various points in the skin to trigger the release of natural painkillers in the body and stimulate increased blood flow.

Biofeedback makes use of electrodes attached to the skin to help people focus and control certain involuntary functions to alleviate pain and achieve relaxation.

Guided imagery also helps diabetic patients achieve relaxation by directing the imagination to account for peaceful and tranquil scenes. By focusing on these, attention to pain is diverted and forgotten.

Progressive muscle relaxation, or PMR for short, is a 2-step technique developed in the 1930's by Jacobson.

It enables patients to tense certain muscles in the body and to concentrate on these muscles as the tension is slowly released to achieve a state of relaxation.

Practice helps patients differentiate between tensed and relaxed muscles, and in turn gives them mental control to relax tensed muscles in the body.

However, a patient should get proper consultation before considering PMR to avoid the risk of aggravating pain in the joints or muscles, especially if he or she has a history of back problems or other grave physical injuries.

PMR if recommended, should be practiced at least twice every day for a week before attempting shortened versions of the entire procedure.

To experience complete satisfaction, it is best to practice the procedure in a place where there are no distractions, not even musical accompaniment. Dress for convenience to facilitate ease of movement.

Do practice before meals to avoid constricting the digestive system from functioning effectively. It's wise to abstain from vices to avoid any unpleasant situations.

A chair would offer comfort, but there is a tendency that sleep may prevail if practicing PMR while lying down. Falling asleep before completion of the full procedure however, does not indicate failure.

If anything, credit yourself for the effort. If you must practice at night on bed when sleep is easy to come over, plan on doing so before completion of the cycle. Add this to the basic cycle.

Rise up slowly after completion of a session to avoid the blood pressure from falling drastically due to sudden standing-up movements. This may even cause one to faint.

Diaphragmatic breathing or yoga can also help diabetic patients relax. They can do this in addition to PMR to completely relax their body and mind.

Individuals with Type 1 diabetes are required to take insulin injections. The number of injections for each patient differs depending on the type of insulin prescribed.

The types of insulin are grouped according to speed and length of efficacy. These include rapid-acting, short-acting, intermediate acting, long-acting and pre-mixed insulin.

The type of insulin prescribed by the doctor takes into account the patient's age, response to insulin, lifestyle choices, frequency of checking blood sugar level, diabetes plan goals and willingness for multiple shots.

The doctor will demonstrate how to administer the injections and guide the patient on how to perform urine or blood tests to check blood sugar.

There are several ways insulin can be injected through the skin.

Aside from syringes, insulin pens are also used, which contain pre-filled cartridges, the contents of which are injected via a fine needle. Using high-pressure air mechanism, jet injectors spray insulin through the skin. Pumps, on the other hand, supply insulin via a catheter attached under the abdomen skin.

With practice, the patients can safely conduct these tests. Recording the measurement of blood sugar on a separate diary or notebook can help patients determine which foods and activities work best for them.

For Type 2 diabetics, there is no need to take insulin injections. Your pancreas is able to produce it, but the substance being produced does not do its job or the amount being produced is too much.

Just maintain a healthy lifestyle.

If maintaining a healthy lifestyle fails to normalize your blood glucose, your doctor might give you some tablets with the purpose of either increasing your insulin production, or helping your body use insulin more effectively or slowing down the cell absorption of the insulin being produced.

Your doctor might resort to prescribing insulin injections if the tablets fail to normalize your blood sugar.

It has been shown that *weight loss surgery* helps to normalize blood sugar levels. This is particularly true for Type 2 diabetes. The amount of lost weight is proportional to the improvement of blood sugar level.

If you will undergo this surgery, there is still the possibility of gaining back the lost weight afterwards.

When this occurs, the diabetes symptoms will reappear. But if you will be successful in maintaining the right weight, there will come a time when you will no longer have to take your medicines.

There are different types of surgery for effective weight loss. Some of these shrink the stomach size to quickly induce a full feeling after meals.

Others change the absorption limit of calories and nutrients by the body. Some even do both.

Gastric bypass, gastric sleeve, gastric band, and bilio-pancreatic diversion are some of the options for weight loss surgery.

In gastric bypass, the top part of the stomach is divided from the rest of it by making a small pouch.

Food goes into this pouch then bypasses the top part of the small intestine. The patient will feel full faster; however there is only less absorption of calories and nutrients.

In gastric sleeve, a major part of the stomach is removed to give the person a fuller feeling after small meals.

This procedure also significantly lowers ghrelin, the hormone that induces hunger.

In adjustable gastric band, an inflatable band is inserted around the top of the stomach to make a small pouch.

A port is used to adjust the gastric band post-surgery to make one full after food passes into this small pouch.

Bilio-pancreatic diversion, is not commonly done as it poses a lot of complications. In this procedure, a large section of the stomach is removed and attached to the large intestine.

While many of these surgeries are effective when it comes to weight loss, there are also several considerations such as the risks and complications involved.

It is best for diabetics to refer to all options available before making a decision. Some doctors will advise to lose weight before considering such procedures.

What about the treatment that utilize *stem cells* and *islet cell transplantation*? Unfortunately, stem cells are showing a good promise, but as of the present, they are not yet considered a treatment.

However, medical experts had some degree of success using stem cells in Type1 diabetes.

Islet cell transplantation is also very promising, having shown that it can improve the quality of life of a patient.

Provided by a donor, islet cells can perceive the rising and lowering of blood sugar levels.

Depending on the level that they can sense, they produce appropriate amounts of insulin. This function allows the recipient to be more flexible in making his meals.

Further, the recipient becomes less prone to long-term diabetes complications that include eye damage, nerve degeneration, heart attack, stroke, and kidney problems. There is still a setback for this treatment.

One who had undergone islet cell transplantation will have to take medicines designed to prevent the body from rejecting the cells from the donor and they have to take these medicines for the rest of his life.

The last medical treatment option is a *pancreas transplant*. This is usually advised for those whose kidneys have already been seriously damaged.

The patient must also take some medicines for life to prevent rejection of the donor pancreas.

Remember that your body is unique and every single day, it is in a different condition compared its condition yesterday.

You cannot just copy the things that one successful diabetic is doing.

You need to have a deep understanding of how your own body reacts to different kinds of foods, different emotional states, different treatments and different physical activities.

As you go along and take note of what is happening inside, you will discover more and more about your body and about your sickness. You can have full control of your condition if you know much.

What you do will largely determine the quality of life you can live. Live your life to its fullest despite the odds. Be happy in spite of everything.

BONUS CHAPTER

Staying Positive

While it's important to learn and relearn everything a diabetic can about his or her condition and how certain lifestyle habits complicate the condition, it is equally important to have a positive attitude.

The effects of a diabetes plan can be best appreciated when a diabetic clears his or her mind of self-doubt and self-pity.

No good is going to come out of such a mental state. Worse, it affects one emotionally and this in turn can increase blood sugar level – the very thing that any doctor or patient needs to avoid to prevent further complications.

Many diabetics get caught up in their condition that they forget to pay attention to the positive things in life. The trick is to think about being the best you can be and doing the best you can do for yourself.

With discipline and commitment, you can be your own best friend -always making sure that you are in the best of health and avoiding situations that cause any harm to your body and condition.

Diabetics can be fun and spontaneous too without having to compromise the diabetes plan. To help break the monotony of the plan, they can make a list of all the things they want to do for themselves.

Of course, making the time for those things comes after. Some diabetics start by fixing what they can at home.

Whether it be fixing the closet to make more space or picking up the unused stuff from different corners of the home to have a garage sale.

There are many things that one can possibly do at home. All it takes is a little creativity and determination.

If staying at home is not someone's idea of having quality me-time, he or she can manage a light jog in the park or visit the nearby museum.

Of course, he or she shouldn't end up eating a box of chocolates from the nearest confectionery or coffee-house.

Giving in to impulses and urges makes it harder for diabetics. One should learn to indulge in moderation, with the responsibility to record every cheat activity in the diary so that the doctor can advise or approve.

Then there is another way for diabetics to take things off their mind. This of course involves doing something nice for someone else.

It's hard to think of one's own problems when he or she is involved in making things easier for another person. In any part of the city, there are several opportunities and platforms to help the under-privileged and marginalized.

A search on Google or inquiring through peers can give someone a glimpse of the many volunteering opportunities available.

Some of these involve bonding with street kids, taking care of kids with special needs or elderly people, or even an ongoing environmental campaign.

Living with diabetes is not living with a disability.

Sure, there may be violent fluctuations in blood sugar level triggered by emotional stress or physical exertion, intake, medications, even the time of the day. However, if these are anticipated and accepted, one can still be in charge of his life.

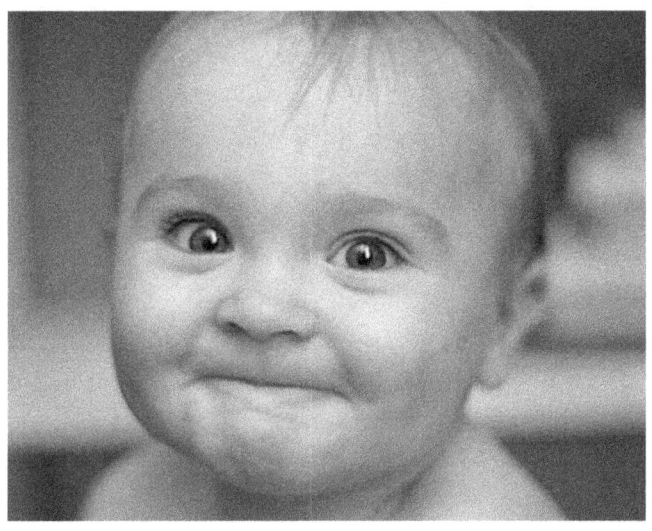

Conclusion

Thank you again for downloading this book!

I hope this book was able to help you to know more about diabetes and realize that you are not at its mercy.

Take seriously the pieces of advice that you have read throughout the book and you can live life just as normally as the next person.

The next step is to make a management plan and follow it religiously.

As soon as you see the good results, be kind enough to share what you have learned to others who are on the same boat. Tell them there is hope for everyone.

Finally, if you enjoyed this book, then I'd like to ask you a favor. Would you be kind enough to leave a review for this book on Amazon? It'd be greatly appreciated!

Please leave a review for this book on Amazon!

Thank you and good luck!